FLAVORS FOR LIFE:

A Diabetes-Friendly Cookbook

BY

BRADLEY M. KEY

DISCLAIMER

TABLE OF CONTENTS

INTRODUCTION

Welcome to 'Flavors for Life: A Diabetes-Friendly Cookbook,' where we embark on a culinary journey designed to empower and inspire those living with diabetes. In this cookbook, we embrace the belief that managing diabetes shouldn't mean sacrificing the joy of delicious, satisfying meals. Instead, it's an opportunity to explore the rich tapestry of flavors, textures, and ingredients that contribute to a well-balanced, healthy lifestyle. In the pages that follow, we unravel the intricate relationship between food and diabetes management, offering a treasure trove of recipes and culinary wisdom crafted specifically for those seeking to strike a harmonious balance between their love for food and their health needs. From hearty breakfasts to sumptuous dinners, from delightful snacks to indulgent desserts, we've carefully curated an array of delectable dishes that cater to diverse tastes and dietary requirements.

Moreover, this cookbook isn't just a collection of recipes. It's a comprehensive guide enriched with valuable insights, practical tips, and nutritional information, all aimed at enhancing your culinary prowess while navigating the intricacies of diabetes management. Join us as we embark on a fulfilling journey, one that celebrates the flavors of life while honoring the path to a healthier, more vibrant future. Let's savor each moment and every bite, relishing the joy of nourishing our bodies and tantalizing our taste buds, all while embracing the delicious potential of diabetes-friendly cooking. Bradley's journey through the realm of diabetes began with uncertainty, but it swiftly transformed into a tale of resilience, discovery, and triumph. When he received the diagnosis, he was apprehensive, fearful of the implications and limitations that diabetes might impose upon his life. But with the unwavering support of his loved ones and the guidance of his healthcare team, he embarked on a quest to conquer diabetes through the power of nutrition.

Armed with determination, Bradley delved into the world of diabetes-friendly nutrition. He educated himself on the significance of low-glycemic index foods, mindful portion control, and balanced meal planning. As he embraced this newfound knowledge, he gradually unlocked the alchemy of transforming his diet into a symphony of wholesome, nourishing ingredients. Bradley's kitchen became his sanctuary, where he concocted culinary masterpieces infused with vibrant flavors and nourishing nutrients. He reveled in the art of crafting hearty salads bursting with colorful vegetables, grilled entrees adorned with aromatic herbs, and decadent yet diabetes-friendly desserts that teased the palate without jeopardizing his well-being. Day by day, Bradley witnessed the transformative power of his nutritional choices. His energy levels soared, his blood sugar levels stabilized, and his overall well-being radiated with newfound vitality. With each passing moment, he savored the delights of savoring meals that not only tantalized his taste buds but also served as allies in his battle against diabetes.

As time unfurled its tapestry, Bradley's resilience and dedication bore fruit. His health improved, and he discovered a newfound sense of empowerment through the agency of his dietary choices. With the compassionate support of his healthcare team and the embrace of a diabetes-friendly culinary lifestyle, Bradley emerged victorious in his quest to conquer diabetes. His journey exemplified the transformative potential of nutrition, proving that with the right dietary approach, one could weave a narrative of vitality, triumph, and savory fulfillment despite the challenges posed by diabetes.

1.1 Understanding Carbohydrates: Empowering Healthy Choices

Understanding the role of carbohydrates is an essential aspect of managing diabetes through nutrition. Carbohydrates have a direct impact on blood sugar levels, making it crucial for individuals with diabetes to discern between

various types of carbohydrates and make informed choices about their consumption.
Bradley's Journey:
Bradley, upon receiving his diabetes diagnosis, faced the daunting task of navigating the intricacies of carbohydrate management. Initially overwhelmed by the myriad of options and conflicting information surrounding carbohydrates, he sought guidance from a registered dietitian specializing in diabetes care. With the dietitian's support, Bradley delved into the realms of healthy carbohydrates. He learned to differentiate between refined carbohydrates — found in sugary snacks and processed foods — and wholesome, complex carbohydrates abundant in whole grains, legumes, and fresh fruits. Over time, he discovered how incorporating more fiber-rich, slow-digesting carbohydrates into his meals led to more stable blood sugar levels and a sustained sense of energy throughout the day. Driven by newfound knowledge and culinary curiosity, Bradley embarked on a culinary adventure, experimenting with a diverse array of nutrient-dense, carb-smart foods. He

savored the earthy sweetness of roasted root vegetables, reveled in the nutty wholesomeness of quinoa, and found delight in ripe, succulent berries that added a burst of natural sweetness to his meals without alarming his blood sugar levels. Through diligent practice and guidance from his healthcare team, Bradley gained confidence in managing his carbohydrate intake. He came to appreciate the intricate dance between carbohydrates, insulin, and his body's response, recognizing that by making mindful choices, he could savor the pleasures of a diverse, well-balanced diet without compromising his health.

Key Points:

Understanding carbohydrates empowered Bradley to make informed choices in his dietary journey. It allowed him to prioritize nutrient-rich, slow-digesting carbohydrates, enabling him to maintain a more stable blood sugar profile while relishing the pleasures of wholesome, satisfying meals. By embracing healthier carbohydrate sources, he was able to transform his relationship with food, savoring the richness of flavors and the vitality of nourishing, diabetes-friendly ingredients. This story illustrates the transformative potential of carbohydrate awareness in the context of diabetes management. It underscores the significance of informed decision-making and the capacity for individuals like Bradley to navigate the complexities of carbohydrate consumption, ultimately paving the way for healthier, more mindful dietary choices. By internalizing the lessons of carbohydrate awareness, individuals with diabetes can embark on a similar journey of nutritional empowerment, transforming their relationship with food, and enhancing their overall well-being through the thoughtful management of carbohydrate intake.

1.2 Tips for Healthy Eating with Diabetes

Eating healthily is of paramount importance for individuals living with diabetes. A balanced, nutritious diet plays a pivotal role in managing blood sugar levels, promoting overall well-being, and reducing the risk of complications associated with diabetes. The following tips are designed to empower individuals with diabetes to make informed dietary choices and cultivate healthier eating habits:

1. **Embrace a Balanced Plate:** Structuring meals around a balanced plate can help regulate blood sugar levels. Aim to fill half of your plate with non-starchy vegetables and divide the remaining half between lean protein and whole grains or starchy vegetables.

2. **Understand Carbohydrates**: Carbohydrates have a substantial impact on blood sugar levels. Learn to identify healthy carbohydrates, such as whole grains, legumes,

and fresh fruits, and limit your intake of refined carbohydrates and added sugars.

3. **Be Mindful of Portion Sizes:** Portion control is crucial for managing blood sugar. Keeping an eye on portion sizes can help prevent overeating and ensure a steady release of glucose into the bloodstream.

4. **Select Healthy Fats:** Opt for heart-healthy unsaturated fats, such as those found in avocados, nuts, seeds, and olive oil. Limit the consumption of saturated and trans fats, which can contribute to cardiovascular risk factors.

5. **Prioritize Lean Proteins:** Incorporate lean sources of protein into your meals, such as poultry, fish, tofu, legumes, and low-fat dairy products. Protein can aid in satiety and assist in stabilizing blood sugar levels.

6. **Favor Fiber-Rich Foods**: Foods high in fiber, including vegetables, fruits, whole grains, and legumes, can help regulate blood sugar

levels, improve digestive health, and contribute to a sense of fullness.

7. **Mindful Eating Practices:** Engage in mindful eating by savoring each bite, eating slowly, and being attuned to hunger and satiety cues. Mindful eating can prevent overeating and promote a healthier relationship with food.

8. **Stay Hydrated:** Adequate hydration is vital for individuals with diabetes. Aim to drink plenty of water throughout the day, as it aids in regulating blood sugar levels and supports overall bodily functions.

9. **Monitor and Adjust:** Regularly monitor your blood sugar levels and be responsive to any fluctuations. Work closely with healthcare professionals to make necessary adjustments to your diet and medication regimen based on these readings.

10. **Seek Professional Guidance:** Consult a registered dietitian or nutritionist with expertise in diabetes management. They can provide

personalized guidance on meal planning, carbohydrate counting, and dietary strategies tailored to your specific needs.

11. **Cultivate Consistency:** Strive for dietary consistency by adhering to regular meal times and choosing a variety of nutrient-dense foods. Consistent eating habits can help stabilize blood sugar levels and support overall metabolic health.

12. **Be Informed and Adventurous:** Stay informed about the nutritional content of foods, and don't be afraid to experiment with new recipes and ingredients that align with your dietary requirements. Variety and culinary exploration can inject excitement and diversity into your diabetes-friendly meals.

By incorporating these tips into your daily routine and embracing a conscious, health-oriented approach to nutrition, you can effectively manage diabetes while savoring the pleasures of wholesome, satisfying meals.

.

CHAPTER 2: BREAKFAST OPTIONS

2.1 Low Glycemic Index Breakfast Ideas

1. **Greek Yogurt Parfait**: Layer Greek yogurt with fresh berries (such as strawberries, blueberries, or raspberries), and a sprinkle of chopped nuts (such as almonds or walnuts). This combination provides a balanced mix of protein, healthy fats, and low-GI carbohydrates.

2. **Oatmeal with Nuts and Seeds:** Prepare a bowl of steel-cut oats or old-fashioned rolled oats and top it with a handful of nuts (e.g., almonds, pecans) and seeds (e.g., chia seeds, flaxseeds). This breakfast is rich in fiber, provides sustained energy, and has a low glycemic load.

3. **Vegetable Omelette**: Whip up an omelette using a variety of colorful vegetables such as bell peppers, spinach, tomatoes, and onions. Vegetables are naturally low in carbohydrates and can slow down the release of glucose into the bloodstream, making this a great low-GI option.

4. **Avocado Toast on Whole Grain Bread:** Mash ripe avocado onto a slice of whole grain bread and top it with a sprinkle of black pepper and a dash of lemon juice. Whole grain bread offers complex carbohydrates, while avocado provides healthy fats and fiber, resulting in a low-GI breakfast choice.

5. **Chia Seed Pudding:** Combine chia seeds with unsweetened almond milk or coconut milk, and allow the mixture to thicken in the refrigerator overnight. In the morning, top it with a few slices of fresh fruit (e.g., kiwi, berries) for a nutrient-packed, low-GI breakfast.

6. **Cottage Cheese and Fruit**: Enjoy a serving of cottage cheese paired with a small portion of fresh fruits such as melon, peaches, or berries. Cottage cheese is high in protein and low in carbohydrates, while the fruits provide natural sweetness and fiber.

7. **Smoothie with Greens and Berries**: Blend together spinach, kale, or other leafy greens with a small portion of berries, a scoop of protein powder, and unsweetened almond milk. This smoothie option is rich in fiber, vitamins, and antioxidants, offering a low-GI breakfast alternative.

8. **Quinoa Breakfast Bowl:** Cook quinoa and serve it with a mix of nuts, seeds, and a small amount of dried or fresh fruit (such as apricots or cranberries). Quinoa is a complex carbohydrate with a lower glycemic index than many other grains, and when combined with protein and healthy fats, it makes for a balanced and low-GI breakfast choice.

These breakfast ideas provide both variety and nutrients, while also being mindful of their impact on blood sugar levels. By incorporating these low glycemic index options into their morning routine, individuals can kickstart their day with sustained energy and metabolic stability, aligning with their goals of diabetes management and overall well-being.

2.2 Healthy Smoothies And Fruit Parfaits

Healthy Smoothies and preparation for Diabetics:

1. **Green Smoothie:**
   - **Ingredients:**
     - 1 cup spinach or kale
     - 1 small cucumber
     - 1 green apple (cored and sliced)
     - 1 tablespoon fresh lemon juice
     - 1/2-inch fresh ginger (peeled)
     - 1/2 to 1 cup water or coconut water

- **Preparation:**
    - Blend all the ingredients until smooth. If needed, add more liquid to achieve the desired consistency. This smoothie is high in fiber and low in sugar, making it a great choice for individuals managing diabetes.

2. **Berry and Chia Smoothie:**
  - **Ingredients:**
    - 1/2 cup mixed berries (such as blueberries, raspberries, strawberries)
    - 1 tablespoon chia seeds
    - 1/2 cup unsweetened almond milk
    - 1/2 cup Greek yogurt (unsweetened)
    - 1/2 teaspoon vanilla extract (optional)
  - **Preparation:**
    - Combine all the ingredients in a blender and blend until smooth. The chia seeds add fiber and healthy fats while the berries provide antioxidants and natural sweetness.

3. **Avocado and Spinach Smoothie:**
  - **Ingredients:**
    - 1/2 ripe avocado

- 1 cup spinach
- 1 small banana (optional for sweetness)
- 1/2 cup unsweetened almond milk
- 1 tablespoon flaxseeds
- **Preparation:**
- Blend all the ingredients until creamy. The healthy fats from the avocado and the fiber from spinach make this a satisfying and low-glycemic smoothie option.

Fruit Parfaits for Diabetics:

1. **Greek Yogurt and Berry Parfait:**
   - **Ingredients:**
     - 1 cup Greek yogurt (unsweetened)
     - 1/2 cup mixed berries
     - 2 tablespoons chopped nuts (e.g., almonds, walnuts)
   - **Preparation:**
     - In a glass, layer the Greek yogurt, mixed berries, and chopped nuts. Repeat the layers if desired. The protein from the yogurt and the fiber from the berries and nuts make this a balanced and diabetes-friendly parfait.

2. **Chia Seed Pudding Parfait:**
   - **Ingredients:**
     - 3 tablespoons chia seeds
     - 1 cup unsweetened almond milk or coconut milk
     - 1/2 teaspoon vanilla extract
     - 1/2 cup sliced strawberries or kiwi
   - **Preparation:**
     - Mix chia seeds, almond milk, and vanilla extract in a bowl, then refrigerate for a few hours or overnight to allow it to thicken. In a glass, layer the chia seed pudding with the sliced fruits. Chia seeds are rich in fiber and protein, making this a filling and diabetes-friendly option.

3. **Cottage Cheese and Fruit Parfait:**
   - **Ingredients:**
     - 1 cup low-fat cottage cheese
     - 1/2 cup fresh fruit (e.g., peaches, berries)
     - 1 tablespoon chopped nuts (optional)
   - **Preparation:**
     - In a glass, layer the cottage cheese with the fresh fruit and nuts if using. Cottage cheese

provides protein, while the fruit adds natural sweetness and fiber, making it a balanced choice for a diabetic-friendly parfait.

These smoothies and fruit parfaits are designed to be low in added sugars, high in fiber, and balanced with protein and healthy fats, making them suitable for individuals with diabetes. Always consult with a healthcare professional or nutritionist to ensure that these options align with an individual's specific dietary needs and diabetes management plan.

2.3 Whole Grain Pancakes and Waffles

Whole Grain Pancakes:
Ingredients:
- 1 cup whole wheat flour
- 1 tablespoon ground flaxseed
- 1 teaspoon baking powder
- 1/2 teaspoon baking soda
- 1/4 teaspoon salt
- 1 cup buttermilk or plain Greek yogurt
- 1/4 cup unsweetened applesauce
- 1 large egg
- 1 tablespoon honey or a sugar-free sweetener (optional)
- 1 teaspoon vanilla extract
- Cooking spray or a small amount of oil for the skillet

Preparation:
1. In a large bowl, whisk together the whole wheat flour, ground flaxseed, baking powder, baking soda, and salt.

2. In a separate bowl, combine the buttermilk or Greek yogurt, unsweetened applesauce, egg, honey or sweetener if using, and vanilla extract.

3. Pour the wet ingredients into the dry ingredients and stir until just combined. Do not overmix.

4. Preheat a non-stick skillet or griddle over medium heat and lightly coat it with cooking spray or oil.

5. Pour 1/4 cup of batter onto the skillet for each pancake.

6. Cook until bubbles form on the surface of the pancake, then flip and cook until golden brown on the other side.

7. Serve with a small amount of sugar-free syrup, fresh berries, or a dollop of Greek yogurt.

Whole Grain Waffles:

Ingredients:
- 1 1/2 cups whole wheat flour
- 2 tablespoons ground flaxseed
- 2 teaspoons baking powder

- 1/2 teaspoon baking soda
- 1/4 teaspoon salt
- 1 3/4 cups buttermilk or plain Greek yogurt
- 1/4 cup unsweetened applesauce
- 2 large eggs
- 2 tablespoons honey or a sugar-free sweetener (optional)
- 1 teaspoon vanilla extract
- Cooking spray or a small amount of oil for the waffle maker

Preparation:

1. In a large bowl, whisk together the whole wheat flour, ground flaxseed, baking powder, baking soda, and salt.

2. In a separate bowl, combine the buttermilk or Greek yogurt, unsweetened applesauce, eggs, honey or sweetener if using, and vanilla extract.

3. Pour the wet ingredients into the dry ingredients and stir until just combined. Do not overmix.

4. Preheat the waffle maker and lightly coat it with cooking spray or oil.

5. Pour the recommended amount of batter onto the waffle maker, close the lid, and cook according to the manufacturer's Preparations.
6. Serve with a small amount of sugar-free syrup, fresh fruit, or a dollop of Greek yogurt.

These whole grain pancake and waffle recipes incorporate fiber-rich whole wheat flour and flaxseed, which can help to slow down the absorption of carbohydrates, thereby potentially leading to a more gradual rise in blood sugar levels. However, it's essential for individuals with diabetes to monitor their blood sugar levels and consult with their healthcare provider or a registered dietitian to ensure that these recipes align with their overall dietary plan.

CHAPTER 3: LUNCH AND DINNER RECIPES

3.1 Delicious Salads and Dressings

Salad Ideas:

1. **Greek Salad with Chicken:**
   - Ingredients:
     - Mixed greens (e.g., spinach, romaine lettuce)
     - Grilled chicken breast
     - Cucumber, cherry tomatoes, red onion, Kalamata olives
     - Feta cheese (in moderation)
     - Optional: a sprinkle of chopped almonds

2. **Quinoa and Vegetable Salad:**
   - Ingredients:
     - Cooked quinoa
     - Mixed vegetables (e.g., bell peppers, cherry tomatoes, cucumber)

- Fresh herbs (e.g., parsley, mint)
    - Lemon juice and a small amount of olive oil for dressing
    - Optional: crumbled feta cheese

3. **Spinach and Berry Salad:**
  - Ingredients:
    - Fresh baby spinach
    - Mixed berries (e.g., strawberries, blueberries, raspberries)
    - Sliced almonds or pecans
    - Goat cheese (in moderation)
    - Balsamic vinaigrette or a simple olive oil and vinegar dressing

4. **Tuna and White Bean Salad:**
  - Ingredients:
    - Canned tuna
    - White beans (e.g., cannellini beans)
    - Mixed greens
    - Sliced red onion, cherry tomatoes
    - Lemon juice and olive oil for dressing

Diabetic-Friendly Salad Dressings:
1. **Lemon-Tahini Dressing:**
- Ingredients:
    - 3 tablespoons tahini
    - 2-3 tablespoons fresh lemon juice
    - 1 clove garlic, minced
    - 1 tablespoon water
    - Salt and pepper to taste

2. **Greek Yogurt and Herb Dressing:**
- Ingredients:
    - 1/2 cup plain Greek yogurt
    - 2 tablespoons chopped fresh herbs (e.g., dill, parsley, chives)
    - 1 tablespoon lemon juice
    - Salt and pepper to taste

3. **Balsamic Vinaigrette with Dijon:**
- Ingredients:
    - 3 tablespoons balsamic vinegar
    - 1 tablespoon Dijon mustard
    - 1/4 cup olive oil
    - 1-2 teaspoons honey or a sugar-free sweetener (optional)

- Salt and pepper to taste

4. **Orange and Ginger Dressing:**
   - Ingredients:
     - 3 tablespoons fresh orange juice
     - 1 teaspoon grated fresh ginger
     - 1 tablespoon olive oil
     - 1 teaspoon honey or a sugar-free sweetener
     - Salt and pepper to taste

These salad and dressing options emphasize fresh produce, lean proteins, healthy fats, and complex carbohydrates, all of which contribute to balanced, diabetes-friendly meals. It's crucial for individuals with diabetes to consider portion sizes and focus on the overall composition of their meals for optimal blood sugar management. Always consult with a healthcare professional or a registered dietitian to tailor these options to specific dietary needs and diabetes management goals.

3.2 Flavorful Soup and Stew Recipes

Vegetable and Lentil Soup:
Ingredients:
- 1 cup dried green or brown lentils, rinsed
- 1 tablespoon olive oil
- 1 onion, diced
- 2 carrots, diced
- 2 stalks celery, diced
- 3 cloves garlic, minced
- 1 teaspoon ground cumin
- 1 teaspoon ground coriander
- 6 cups low-sodium vegetable or chicken broth
- 1 can (14 oz) diced tomatoes
- 2 cups chopped kale or spinach
- Salt and pepper to taste
- Fresh lemon juice for serving

Preparation:
1. In a large pot, heat the olive oil over medium heat. Add the onion, carrots, and celery, and cook until softened, about 5 minutes.

2. Add the garlic, cumin, and coriander, and cook for another minute until fragrant.
3. Stir in the lentils, broth, and diced tomatoes. Bring the soup to a boil, then reduce the heat and let it simmer for about 30-40 minutes or until the lentils are tender.
4. Add the chopped kale or spinach and cook for an additional 5 minutes until wilted.
5. Season with salt, pepper, and a squeeze of fresh lemon juice before serving.

Turkey and Vegetable Stew:
Ingredients:
- 1 tablespoon olive oil
- 1 pound lean turkey breast, cut into cubes
- 1 onion, diced
- 2 carrots, sliced
- 2 parsnips, sliced
- 2 stalks celery, sliced
- 3 cloves garlic, minced
- 1 teaspoon dried thyme
- 1 teaspoon dried rosemary
- 4 cups low-sodium chicken broth
- 1 can (14 oz) white beans, drained and rinsed

- Salt and pepper to taste
- Chopped fresh parsley for garnish

Preparation:
1. In a large pot, heat the olive oil over medium heat. Add the cubed turkey breast and cook until browned on all sides. Remove the turkey from the pot and set it aside.
2. Add the onion, carrots, parsnips, and celery to the pot, and cook until the vegetables start to soften, about 5-7 minutes.
3. Stir in the garlic, thyme, and rosemary, and cook for another minute.
4. Return the browned turkey to the pot, then pour in the chicken broth. Bring the stew to a simmer and let it cook for about 20-25 minutes or until the vegetables are tender and the turkey is cooked through.
5. Add the white beans and cook for an additional 5 minutes to heat through. Season with salt and pepper, and garnish with chopped fresh parsley before serving.

These soup and stew recipes are rich in fiber, lean protein, and an array of vegetables, making them nutritious and suitable for individuals managing diabetes. It's important to consider portion sizes and carbohydrate content when incorporating these recipes into a diabetic meal plan. As always, it's recommended to consult with a healthcare professional or a registered dietitian to ensure these recipes align with individual dietary needs and diabetes management goals.

3.3 Low-carb Pasta and Grain Bowls:

These recipes are designed to provide balanced nutrition while keeping carbohydrate content in check.

Low-Carb Pasta Recipe: Zucchini Noodles with Pesto

Ingredients:
- 4 medium zucchinis
- 2 tablespoons olive oil
- 2 cloves garlic, minced
- Salt and pepper to taste

- 1/4 cup pesto sauce (store-bought or homemade)

Preparations:

1. Using a spiralizer or a vegetable peeler, create zucchini noodles (zoodles) from the zucchinis.
2. Heat olive oil in a large skillet over medium heat. Add minced garlic and sauté for 1-2 minutes.
3. Add the zucchini noodles to the skillet. Sauté for 2-3 minutes until the zoodles are tender but still slightly crisp.
4. Season with salt and pepper to taste.
5. Turn off the heat and stir in the pesto sauce until the zoodles are evenly coated.
6. Serve the zucchini noodles with an additional dollop of pesto if desired.

Low-Carb Grain Bowl Recipe: Cauliflower Rice and Grilled Chicken Bowl

Ingredients:
- 2 cups cauliflower rice
- 1 teaspoon olive oil
- 1 teaspoon dried oregano
- Salt and pepper to taste
- 4 oz. grilled chicken breast, sliced
- 1/4 cup cherry tomatoes, halved
- 1/4 cup cucumber, diced
- 1/4 cup bell peppers, sliced
- 1/4 cup feta cheese, crumbled
- 2 tablespoons balsamic vinaigrette

Preparations:

1. In a skillet, heat olive oil over medium-high heat. Add cauliflower rice, oregano, salt, and pepper. Sauté for 5-7 minutes, until the cauliflower rice is tender.

2. Transfer the cooked cauliflower rice to a serving bowl.

3. Arrange the grilled chicken slices, cherry tomatoes, cucumber, and bell peppers on top of the cauliflower rice.
4. Sprinkle with crumbled feta cheese and drizzle with balsamic vinaigrette.
5. Toss gently to combine all the ingredients, and enjoy your low-carb grain bowl!

These recipes provide fiber-rich, low-carb alternatives to traditional pasta and grain bowls, helping to manage blood sugar levels and keeping meals delicious and satisfying, even for individuals with diabetes.

Bradley was an avid food lover, with a particular fondness for pasta and hearty grain bowls. However, he faced an unexpected adversary: diabetes. Determined to conquer this challenge, Bradley embarked on a transformative culinary journey that would change his life. Bradley sought out nutritious and innovative recipes to manage his diabetes while still savoring delicious meals. As he delved into the world of low-carb cooking, he discovered the remarkable versatility of zucchini noodles and cauliflower rice. Intrigued by the prospects of these healthier alternatives, he set out to revolutionize his dietary habits. Armed with fresh zucchinis, a trusty spiralizer, and a head of cauliflower, Bradley embraced his new culinary mission. He meticulously crafted zucchini noodles with flavorful pesto, savoring the delicate aroma and satisfying texture. To complement this new dish, he conjured a unique grain bowl brimming with cauliflower rice, grilled chicken, and a vibrant medley of fresh vegetables, crowned with a drizzle of tangy balsamic vinaigrette. With unwavering commitment, Bradley incorporated these low-carb, nutrient-dense recipes into his daily routine. He dedicated himself to savoring the vibrant colors and tantalizing flavors of his newfound culinary creations. Soon, he began to witness a remarkable transformation – his blood sugar levels stabilized, and his energy levels surged. As the days turned into weeks, and the weeks into months, Bradley's steadfast resolve and wholesome culinary choices led to a profound shift in his well-being.

As Bradley embraced his commitment to healthier eating, he discovered a newfound sense of empowerment and vitality. He shared his success with friends and family, regaling them with stories of his culinary adventures, and inspiring them to embark on their own paths toward a healthier lifestyle. Over time, Bradley triumphantly conquered the challenges posed by diabetes, his diligence reflecting in his improved overall health. His zest for life and his passion for flavorful, nutritious cuisine became a beacon of hope and inspiration for others navigating similar journeys.

Through his unwavering commitment to wholesome, low-carb meals, Bradley prevailed over adversity, emerging not just victorious in his battle with diabetes, but as a beacon of inspiration for the transformative power of conscious, healthful choices. And so, Bradley's remarkable journey echoed throughout the town, a testament to the remarkable potential for positive change that lies within the simple pleasure of a well-crafted, nutritious meal.

3.4 Grilled and Baked Entrees with Vegetable Sides

Grilled Lemon Garlic Salmon with Roasted Asparagus

Grilled Lemon Garlic Salmon
Ingredients:
- 4 boneless salmon fillets
- 2 tablespoons olive oil
- 3 cloves garlic, minced
- 2 tablespoons fresh lemon juice
- 1 teaspoon lemon zest
- Salt and pepper to taste
- Fresh dill or parsley for garnish (optional)

Preparations:
1. Preheat a grill to medium-high heat.
2. In a small bowl, whisk together the olive oil, minced garlic, lemon juice, lemon zest, salt, and pepper to create a marinade for the salmon.

3. Place the salmon fillets in a dish and pour the marinade over them. Let them marinate for 20-30 minutes.

4. Grill the salmon fillets for 4-5 minutes on each side, or until they are cooked to your desired degree of doneness.

5. Garnish with fresh dill or parsley before serving.

Roasted Asparagus
Ingredients:
- 1 bunch asparagus, woody ends trimmed
- 2 tablespoons olive oil
- Salt and pepper to taste
- Grated Parmesan cheese (optional)

Preparations:
1. Preheat the oven to 400°F (200°C).

2. Place the asparagus on a baking sheet. Drizzle with olive oil, and season with salt and pepper.

3. Toss the asparagus to ensure it's evenly coated with the oil and seasonings.

4. Roast the asparagus for 10-15 minutes, or until it is tender and slightly browned at the tips.

5. Sprinkle with grated Parmesan cheese if desired before serving.

Baked Lemon Herb Chicken with Steamed Green Beans

Baked Lemon Herb Chicken
Ingredients:
- 4 boneless, skinless chicken breasts
- 3 tablespoons olive oil
- 2 tablespoons fresh lemon juice
- 2 cloves garlic, minced
- 1 teaspoon dried thyme
- 1 teaspoon dried rosemary
- Salt and pepper to taste
- Lemon slices for garnish (optional)

Preparations:
1. Preheat the oven to 375°F (190°C).

2. In a small bowl, whisk together the olive oil, lemon juice, minced garlic, thyme, rosemary,

salt, and pepper to create a marinade for the chicken.

3. Place the chicken breasts in a baking dish and pour the marinade over them. Let them marinate for 30 minutes.

4. Bake the chicken for 25-30 minutes or until the internal temperature reaches 165°F (75°C).

5. Garnish with lemon slices before serving.

Steamed Green Beans

Ingredients:

- 1 pound fresh green beans, trimmed
- 2 tablespoons butter
- 2 cloves garlic, minced
- Salt and pepper to taste
- Lemon zest for garnish (optional)

Preparations:

1. Place the green beans in a steamer basket over boiling water. Cover and steam for 4-5 minutes until they are tender-crisp.

2. In a small skillet, melt the butter, then add the minced garlic. Cook for 1-2 minutes until fragrant.

3. Toss the steamed green beans in the garlic butter, and season with salt and pepper.
4. Garnish with lemon zest before serving.

These recipes offer a delectable combination of grilled and baked entrees paired with delicious vegetable sides, offering a healthy and diabetes-friendly dining experience. Enjoy!

CHAPTER 4. SNACKS AND APPETIZERS

4.1 NUTRITIOUS SNACK IDEAS

For individuals managing diabetes, creating nutritious and satisfying snack options is essential for maintaining stable blood sugar levels. These delicious and diabetes-friendly snack ideas is just right:

1. Greek Yogurt and Berries

Enjoy a serving of plain Greek yogurt topped with fresh berries such as strawberries, blueberries, or raspberries. This snack provides a good balance of protein, healthy fats, and fiber to help keep blood sugar levels stable.

2. Almonds and Clementine

Pair a small handful of almonds with a clementine for a delightful snack that combines healthy fats, protein, and fiber with the natural sweetness of the clementine.

3. **Carrot Sticks and Hummus**

Dip fresh carrot sticks into a portion of hummus for a satisfying and crunchy snack. Carrots are a great source of fiber and nutrients, while hummus provides both protein and healthy fats.

4. **Cottage Cheese and Sliced Cucumbers**

Combine cottage cheese with fresh sliced cucumbers for a refreshing and protein-rich snack. Cottage cheese offers a good source of protein, while cucumbers add a refreshing crunch.

5. **Hard-Boiled Eggs with a Sprinkle of Everything Bagel Seasoning**

Enjoy a hard-boiled egg sprinkled with a dash of everything bagel seasoning for a flavorful, protein-packed snack that's quick and easy to prepare.

6. **Avocado with Whole Grain Crackers**

Slice half an avocado and enjoy it with a few whole grain crackers. Avocado provides healthy fats, while whole grain crackers offer fiber and essential nutrients.

7. **Edamame Beans**

Snack on a serving of edamame beans for a plant-based protein snack that's rich in fiber. Simply steam or boil edamame pods and sprinkle with a touch of sea salt.

8. **Tuna Salad Lettuce Wraps**

Prepare a small portion of tuna salad and scoop it into lettuce leaves for a refreshing and protein-rich snack. Be mindful of the amount of mayo and high-carb ingredients you use in your tuna salad for a lower-carb variation.

9. **Sliced Apple with Peanut Butter**

Slice an apple and enjoy it with a dollop of natural peanut butter. The combination of crunchy, sweet apple and creamy peanut butter provides a delightful mix of fiber, healthy fats, and a touch of natural sweetness.

10. **Chia Seed Pudding**

Prepare a small serving of chia seed pudding using unsweetened almond milk, chia seeds, and a touch of vanilla extract. Sweeten with a small amount of natural sweetener or a sprinkle of cinnamon.

These snack ideas offer nutritious and balanced options for individuals managing diabetes, providing a mix of protein, healthy fats, and fiber to help stabilize blood sugar levels and keep you feeling satisfied between meals.

4.2 Vegetable and Hummus Platters:

Creating flavorful and diabetes-friendly vegetable and hummus platters can be both delicious and nutritious! Here are a few ideas for assembling these platters:

Classic Vegetable and Hummus Platter
Ingredients:
- 1 cup hummus (store-bought or homemade)
- 1 cucumber, sliced
- 2 carrots, peeled and cut into sticks
- 2 bell peppers, sliced
- 1 cup cherry tomatoes
- 1 cup snap peas
- 2 celery stalks, cut into sticks

Preparations:
1. Arrange the hummus in the center of a large platter or serving dish.
2. Surround the hummus with an assortment of colorful vegetables, such as cucumber slices, carrot sticks, bell pepper slices, cherry tomatoes, snap peas, and celery sticks.
3. For added visual appeal, you can organize the different vegetables in separate sections around the hummus, creating an inviting and vibrant display.

This classic platter offers a diverse mix of crunchy, fresh vegetables along with creamy, protein-rich hummus, providing a satisfying and nutritious snack.

Mediterranean Inspired Vegetable and Hummus Platter

Ingredients:
- 1 1/2 cups hummus (store-bought or homemade)
- 1 cucumber, sliced
- 1 cup cherry tomatoes
- 1/2 cup Kalamata olives
- 4-6 whole roasted red peppers (from a jar)
- 1/2 cup feta cheese, crumbled
- 2 tablespoons extra virgin olive oil
- Freshly chopped parsley for garnish

Preparations:
1. Place the hummus in the center of a large platter.

2. Surround the hummus with cucumber slices, cherry tomatoes, Kalamata olives, and whole roasted red peppers.
3. Sprinkle crumbled feta cheese over the hummus and around the platter.
4. Drizzle extra virgin olive oil over the hummus and the assorted vegetables.
5. Garnish with freshly chopped parsley for a burst of fresh flavor.

This Mediterranean-inspired platter offers a delightful mix of savory and tangy flavors, perfect for a light and satisfying snack.

Spicy Vegetable and Hummus Platter
Ingredients:
- 1 1/2 cups spicy hummus (store-bought or homemade)
- 2 carrots, peeled and cut into sticks
- 2 celery stalks, cut into sticks
- 1 bell pepper, sliced
- 1 cup radishes, halved
- 1/2 cup pickled jalapeños
- 1/4 cup hot sauce (optional, for extra heat)

Preparations:
1. Spread the spicy hummus in the center of a large platter.
2. Arrange the assortment of vegetables around the hummus, including carrot sticks, celery sticks, bell pepper slices, radish halves, and pickled jalapeños.
3. For those who enjoy an extra kick of heat, drizzle hot sauce over the spicy hummus or include it in a small dish on the platter.

This spicier take on the classic hummus platter offers a zesty and bold flavor profile, perfect for those who enjoy a bit of heat in their snacks. These vegetable and hummus platters provide a variety of healthy, diabetes-friendly options, showcasing the versatility and deliciousness of simple, wholesome ingredients. They're great for both solo enjoyment and for sharing with friends and family at gatherings or parties. Enjoy!

4.3 Healthy Dips and Spreads

Creating delicious and diabetes-friendly dips and spreads can open up a world of flavorful and nutritious snack options. Here are some ideas for healthy and satisfying dips and spreads suitable for individuals managing diabetes:

1. **Guacamole**

Ingredients:
- 2 ripe avocados
- 1 small red onion, finely diced
- 1 tomato, diced
- 1 jalapeño, minced (seeds removed for milder flavor)
- 2 tablespoons chopped fresh cilantro
- 1-2 tablespoons lime juice
- Salt and pepper to taste

Preparations:
1. In a medium bowl, mash the avocados to your desired consistency.
2. Stir in the diced red onion, tomato, jalapeño, and fresh cilantro.

3. Add lime juice, salt, and pepper, adjusting to taste.
4. Serve with an assortment of fresh vegetables such as cucumber slices, bell pepper strips, or carrot sticks.

Guacamole offers creamy richness, healthy fats, and a vibrant burst of flavor, making it a delightful and diabetes-friendly dip.

2. **Greek Yogurt Dip**

Ingredients:
- 1 cup plain Greek yogurt
- 1 clove garlic, minced
- 1 tablespoon fresh lemon juice
- 1 teaspoon chopped fresh dill
- Salt and pepper to taste

Preparations:
1. In a small bowl, combine Greek yogurt, minced garlic, lemon juice, and fresh dill.
2. Season with salt and pepper, adjusting to taste.
3. Refrigerate for 30 minutes before serving to allow the flavors to meld.

4. Pair with a variety of fresh vegetables or whole grain pita bread for a nutritious and satisfying snack.

Greek yogurt dip provides a protein-rich and tangy alternative to traditional creamy dips, adding a refreshing element to your snacking.

3. **Roasted Red Pepper Hummus**

Ingredients:

- 1 can (15 oz) chickpeas, drained and rinsed
- 2 roasted red peppers (from a jar), drained and patted dry
- 2 tablespoons tahini
- 2 cloves garlic, minced
- 3 tablespoons lemon juice
- 2 tablespoons extra virgin olive oil
- 1/2 teaspoon ground cumin
- Salt to taste

Preparations:

1. In a food processor, combine chickpeas, roasted red peppers, tahini, minced garlic, lemon juice, extra virgin olive oil, and ground cumin.

2. Process until smooth, adding a little water if needed to achieve the desired consistency.
3. Season with salt, adjusting to taste.
4. Serve with crunchy raw vegetables or whole grain crackers for a delicious and fiber-rich snack.

Roasted red pepper hummus offers a flavorful and fiber-packed dip option that's perfect for dipping or spreading on whole grain toast or wraps.

4. Olive Tapenade

Ingredients:
- 1 cup pitted Kalamata olives
- 2 cloves garlic, minced
- 2 tablespoons capers
- 1 tablespoon fresh lemon juice
- 2 tablespoons chopped fresh parsley
- 3 tablespoons extra virgin olive oil
- Black pepper to taste

Preparations:
1. Place the Kalamata olives, minced garlic, capers, lemon juice, and chopped parsley in a food processor.
2. Pulse the mixture while drizzling in the extra virgin olive oil until it reaches a chunky yet spreadable consistency.
3. Season with black pepper, adjusting to taste.
4. Spread on whole grain crackers or use as a dip for raw vegetable sticks.

Olive tapenade provides savory and piquant spread rich in heart-healthy fats, offering a unique and flavorful option for your snacking needs.

These wholesome dips and spreads are not only delicious but also provide balanced nutrition, making them ideal choices for individuals managing diabetes. Enjoy your snacking with these diabetes-friendly options!

CHAPTER 5: DESSERTS AND TREATS

5.1 Sugar-free and fruit-based desserts for diabetics

Creating delicious, sugar-free, and fruit-based desserts can be both satisfying and suitable for individuals managing diabetes. Here are some delightful and diabetes-friendly dessert ideas that prioritize the natural sweetness of fruits and avoid added sugars:

1. Mixed Berry Parfait

Ingredients:

- 1 cup mixed berries (such as strawberries, blueberries, raspberries)
- 1 cup plain Greek yogurt
- 1 tablespoon chopped nuts (almonds, walnuts, or pecans)

Preparations:

1. In a glass or serving dish, layer mixed berries and plain Greek yogurt.

2. Repeat the layers as desired, ending with a dollop of yogurt on top.
3. Sprinkle chopped nuts over the yogurt for added crunch and healthy fats.

This mixed berry parfait offers a balance of natural sweetness from the berries, creamy richness from the Greek yogurt, and a satisfying crunch from the nuts.

2. **Baked Apples with Cinnamon**

Ingredients:
- 4 apples, cored and halved
- 1 teaspoon ground cinnamon
- 1/2 teaspoon ground nutmeg
- 1 tablespoon chopped unsweetened dried fruit (such as apricots or raisins)
- 1 tablespoon chopped nuts (such as almonds or pecans)

Preparations:
1. Preheat the oven to 350°F (175°C).
2. Place the apple halves in a baking dish.

3. In a small bowl, mix together the ground
cinnamon, ground nutmeg, chopped dried fruit,
and chopped nuts.
4. Sprinkle the cinnamon mixture over the
apple halves.
5. Bake for 20-25 minutes, or until the apples
are tender.
6. Serve the baked apples warm, with a dollop
of Greek yogurt if desired.

Baked apples with cinnamon and a touch of
dried fruit offer a warm, aromatic, and naturally
sweet dessert that's perfect for satisfying
dessert cravings.

3. **Mango Sorbet**

Ingredients:
- 2 ripe mangoes, peeled and diced
- 1-2 tablespoons fresh lime juice

Preparations:
1. Place the diced mangoes and fresh lime juice
in a blender or food processor.

2. Blend until smooth, adding a small amount of water if needed to achieve a sorbet-like consistency.

3. Transfer the mango mixture into a shallow container and freeze for 3-4 hours, stirring occasionally to prevent large ice crystals from forming.

4. Serve scoops of the mango sorbet in bowls or as a refreshing dessert after a satisfying meal.

Mango sorbet offers a lusciously smooth and fruity dessert option without the need for added sugars, providing a cool and refreshing treat.

4. **Berry Chia Seed Pudding**

Ingredients:
- 1/4 cup chia seeds
- 1 cup unsweetened almond milk (or any preferred unsweetened milk)
- 1-2 tablespoons pure vanilla extract
- 1 cup mixed berries (such as strawberries, blueberries, raspberries)

Preparations:
1. In a bowl, mix the chia seeds, unsweetened almond milk, and pure vanilla extract.
2. Refrigerate the mixture for at least 2 hours or overnight, stirring occasionally, until it thickens into a pudding-like consistency.
3. Once the chia pudding has set, layer it with mixed berries in serving dishes.
4. Enjoy the creamy and naturally sweetened chia seed pudding as a guilt-free dessert or snack.

This berry chia seed pudding offers a comforting and nutritious dessert option that's packed with fiber and the natural sweetness of berries.

These sugar-free and fruit-based desserts provide a delightful and satisfying way to indulge in treats without compromising on healthy eating goals. Enjoy these delicious dessert alternatives while managing diabetes and savor the natural sweetness of fruits!

5.2: Light and Tasty baked goods for diabetics

Creating light and tasty baked goods for individuals managing diabetes is definitely possible. Here are some delicious and diabetes-friendly options that prioritize wholesome ingredients and moderation in portion sizes:

1. Almond Flour Blueberry Muffins
Ingredients:
- 2 cups almond flour
- 1/4 cup coconut flour
- 1/2 teaspoon baking soda
- 1/4 teaspoon salt
- 3 large eggs
- 1/4 cup unsweetened almond milk
- 1/4 cup melted coconut oil
- 1/4 cup honey or a sugar-free sweetener of your choice
- 1 teaspoon pure vanilla extract
- 1 cup fresh blueberries

Preparations:

1. Preheat the oven to 350°F (175°C) and line a muffin tin with paper liners.
2. In a large bowl, whisk together the almond flour, coconut flour, baking soda, and salt.
3. In a separate bowl, whisk the eggs, almond milk, melted coconut oil, honey (or sweetener), and vanilla extract until well combined.
4. Gradually add the wet ingredients to the dry ingredients, stirring until just combined.
5. Gently fold in the fresh blueberries.
6. Divide the batter evenly among the muffin cups.
7. Bake for 20-25 minutes, or until the muffins are golden and a toothpick inserted into the center comes out clean.
8. Allow the muffins to cool in the tin for 5 minutes before transferring to a wire rack to cool completely.

These almond flour blueberry muffins offer a delightful balance of wholesome ingredients and natural sweetness, making them a delicious and diabetes-friendly baked treat.

2. **Oatmeal Banana Cookies**

Ingredients:

- 2 ripe bananas, mashed
- 2 cups old-fashioned oats
- 1/4 cup chopped nuts (such as walnuts or almonds)
- 1/4 cup unsweetened shredded coconut
- 1/4 cup raisins or dried cranberries
- 1 teaspoon pure vanilla extract
- 1/2 teaspoon ground cinnamon
- A pinch of salt

Preparations:

1. Preheat the oven to 350°F (175°C) and line a baking sheet with parchment paper.
2. In a bowl, combine the mashed bananas, oats, chopped nuts, shredded coconut, raisins or dried cranberries, vanilla extract, ground cinnamon, and a pinch of salt.
3. Drop spoonfuls of the cookie mixture onto the prepared baking sheet and flatten slightly with the back of a spoon.
4. Bake for 12-15 minutes, or until the cookies are golden and set.

5. Allow the cookies to cool on the baking sheet for a few minutes before transferring to a wire rack to cool completely.

These oatmeal banana cookies provide a chewy and wholesome dessert option without added sugars, offering the natural sweetness of ripe bananas and dried fruits.

3. **Whole Wheat Zucchini Bread Ingredients:**
- 1 1/2 cups whole wheat flour
- 1 teaspoon baking powder
- 1/2 teaspoon baking soda
- 1/2 teaspoon ground cinnamon
- 1/4 teaspoon salt
- 2 eggs
- 1/3 cup olive oil
- 1/2 cup honey or a sugar-free sweetener of your choice
- 1 teaspoon pure vanilla extract
- 1 1/2 cups grated zucchini
- 1/2 cup chopped nuts (such as walnuts or pecans)

Preparations:
1. Preheat the oven to 350°F (175°C) and grease a loaf pan.
2. In a large bowl, whisk together the whole wheat flour, baking powder, baking soda, ground cinnamon, and salt.
3. In a separate bowl, whisk the eggs, olive oil, honey (or sweetener), and vanilla extract until well combined.
4. Gradually add the wet ingredients to the dry ingredients, stirring until just combined.
5. Fold in the grated zucchini and chopped nuts.
6. Pour the batter into the prepared loaf pan.
7. Bake for 50-60 minutes, or until a toothpick inserted into the center comes out clean.
8. Allow the zucchini bread to cool in the pan for 10 minutes before transferring to a wire rack to cool completely.

This whole wheat zucchini bread provides a fiber-rich and naturally sweetened baked good, perfect for a satisfying and wholesome treat.

These light and tasty baked goods prioritize nutrient-dense ingredients and the natural sweetness of fruits, making them suitable choices for individuals managing diabetes who want to indulge in a delightful dessert without compromising their health goals. Enjoy these wholesome and satisfying treats in moderation!

5.3 Indulgent-yet-healthy dessert ideas for diabetics

Indulging in a wholesome and satisfying dessert while managing diabetes is absolutely achievable. Here are a few indulgent yet healthy dessert ideas that prioritize natural sweetness, nutrient-dense ingredients, and mindful portion sizes:

1. **Dark Chocolate-Dipped Strawberries Ingredients:**
- Fresh strawberries, washed and dried
- High-quality dark chocolate (70% cocoa or higher)

Preparations:
1. Line a baking sheet with parchment paper.
2. In a microwave-safe bowl, melt the dark chocolate in 20-second intervals, stirring between each, until smooth and fully melted.
3. Holding a strawberry by the stem, dip it into the melted dark chocolate, allowing any excess chocolate to drip off.
4. Place the chocolate-covered strawberry on the prepared baking sheet.
5. Once all strawberries are dipped, refrigerate the baking sheet for 15-20 minutes, or until the chocolate has set.

Dark chocolate-dipped strawberries offer a delightful combination of juicy sweetness and rich, antioxidant-packed dark chocolate, making them a luscious yet healthful dessert option.

2. Greek Yogurt Parfait with Nuts and Berries

Ingredients:
- Plain Greek yogurt

- Mixed berries (such as blueberries, raspberries, or strawberries)
- Chopped nuts (such as almonds, walnuts, or pistachios)
- Drizzle of honey or a sprinkle of stevia (optional)

Preparations:
1. In a glass or a serving dish, layer plain Greek yogurt with a generous portion of mixed berries.
2. Sprinkle a layer of chopped nuts on top of the berries.
3. Add another layer of yogurt, followed by an additional layer of mixed berries and nuts.
4. Optionally, drizzle a small amount of honey or sprinkle stevia for additional sweetness.
5. Serve immediately and enjoy its creamy and fruity goodness.

This Greek yogurt parfait with nuts and berries offers a delightful blend of protein-packed yogurt, antioxidant-rich berries, and heart-healthy nuts, creating a satisfying and indulgent dessert.

3. **Nutty Baked Apples**
Ingredients:
- Whole apples, such as Granny Smith or Honeycrisp
- Chopped nuts (such as almonds or pecans)
- Ground cinnamon
- 1-2 tablespoons unsweetened shredded coconut
- A sprinkle of nutmeg (optional)
- Dollop of Greek yogurt (optional)

Preparations:
1. Preheat the oven to 375°F (190°C).
2. Core the apples and place them in a baking dish lined with parchment paper.
3. In a small bowl, mix together chopped nuts, ground cinnamon, unsweetened shredded coconut, and nutmeg, if desired.
4. Stuff the apple cores with the nut mixture.
5. Bake for 20-25 minutes, or until the apples are tender and the nut filling is golden.
6. Serve the nutty baked apples warm, optionally accompanied by a dollop of Greek yogurt for a creamy contrast.

Nutty baked apples provide a warm, comforting, and indulgent dessert that's rich in fiber, offering a delightful balance of natural sweetness and nutty goodness.

These options allow for indulgence while staying mindful of managing diabetes. They combine rich flavors, natural sweetness, and nutrient-dense ingredients, providing a delightful way to savor a satisfying dessert without compromising overall health. Enjoy these indulgent-yet-healthy dessert ideas in moderation as part of a balanced lifestyle.

CHAPTER 6: HOLIDAY AND SPECIAL OCCASION MENUS

6.1 Festive recipes for celebration for diabetics

Celebrating with delicious and diabetes-friendly festive recipes is both enjoyable and achievable. Here are some delightful and wholesome recipes perfect for celebrations:

1. Herb-Roasted Turkey Breast with Cranberry Chutney
Herb-Roasted Turkey Breast:
- 3-4 pounds bone-in turkey breast
- 3 tablespoons olive oil
- 1 tablespoon chopped fresh rosemary
- 1 tablespoon chopped fresh thyme
- Salt and pepper to taste

Preparations:

1. Preheat the oven to 350°F (175°C).
2. In a small bowl, mix together the olive oil, chopped rosemary, chopped thyme, salt, and pepper.
3. Rub the herb mixture all over the turkey breast.
4. Place the turkey breast on a roasting rack in a roasting pan and roast for about 20 minutes per pound, or until the internal temperature reaches 165°F (75°C).

Cranberry Chutney:

- 12 ounces fresh or frozen cranberries
- 1/2 cup water
- 1/2 cup sugar-free sweetener
- Zest and juice of 1 orange
- 1/2 teaspoon ground cinnamon
- 1/4 teaspoon ground cloves

Preparations:

1. In a saucepan, combine the cranberries, water, sugar-free sweetener, orange zest and juice, ground cinnamon, and ground cloves.

2. Bring the mixture to a boil, then reduce the heat and simmer for 10-15 minutes, or until the cranberries have burst and the chutney has thickened.

This festive Herb-Roasted Turkey Breast paired with Cranberry Chutney offers a savory and sweet centerpiece perfect for special occasions.

2. Quinoa and Roasted Vegetable Stuffed Bell Peppers

Ingredients:

- 4 large bell peppers, tops removed and seeds discarded
- 1 cup quinoa, rinsed
- 2 cups vegetable or chicken broth
- 2 cups mixed roasted vegetables (such as zucchini, eggplant, bell peppers, and cherry tomatoes)
- 1/2 cup crumbled feta cheese
- 2 tablespoons chopped fresh basil
- Salt and pepper to taste

Preparations:

1. Preheat the oven to 375°F (190°C).

2. In a saucepan, bring the quinoa and broth to a boil. Reduce the heat, cover, and simmer for 15-20 minutes, or until the quinoa is tender and the liquid is absorbed.

3. In a bowl, mix the cooked quinoa, roasted vegetables, feta cheese, chopped fresh basil, salt, and pepper.

4. Stuff the bell peppers with the quinoa and roasted vegetable mixture.

5. Place the stuffed bell peppers in a baking dish, and bake for 25-30 minutes, or until the peppers are tender.

These Quinoa and Roasted Vegetable Stuffed Bell Peppers offer a flavorful and nutritious option for a festive vegetarian main course.

3. **Sugar-Free Pumpkin Cheesecake**
Ingredients:
For the Crust:
- 1 1/2 cups almond flour
- 1/4 cup melted butter
- 1 tablespoon sugar-free sweetener
- 1 teaspoon ground cinnamon

For the Filling:
- 24 ounces cream cheese, softened
- 1 cup sugar-free sweetener
- 1 cup canned pumpkin puree
- 3 large eggs
- 1 teaspoon vanilla extract
- 1 teaspoon ground cinnamon
- 1/2 teaspoon ground nutmeg
- 1/4 teaspoon ground cloves

Preparations:
1. Preheat the oven to 325°F (160°C).
2. In a bowl, mix together the almond flour, melted butter, sugar-free sweetener, and ground cinnamon for the crust. Press the

mixture into the bottom of a greased 9-inch springform pan.

3. In a large bowl, beat the cream cheese and sugar-free sweetener until smooth. Add the pumpkin puree, eggs, vanilla extract, ground cinnamon, ground nutmeg, and ground cloves, and beat until well combined.

4. Pour the filling over the crust and smooth the top.

5. Bake for 45-50 minutes, or until the center is almost set.

6. Allow the cheesecake to cool, then refrigerate for at least 4 hours or overnight before serving.

This Sugar-Free Pumpkin Cheesecake offers a decadent and satisfying dessert option perfect for festive occasions. These recipes offer both flavor and nutrition, making them ideal for celebrating without compromising health goals. Enjoy these festive recipes as part of a joyful and wholesome celebration.

6.2 Tips for eating well during festivities for diabetics

Eating well and enjoying festive occasions, while managing diabetes, is both achievable and important. Here are some tips for individuals with diabetes to navigate festive occasions without compromising their health goals:

1. Plan and Prepare Ahead

- Planning ahead can help in making healthier choices. If you know the menu in advance, you can plan your meals and snacks accordingly to balance your carbohydrate intake.

2. Monitor Portion Sizes

- Be mindful of portion sizes, especially when it comes to carbohydrate-rich foods and desserts. Using smaller plates and utensils may help with portion control.

3. Focus on Fiber-Rich Foods

- Including fiber-rich foods such as vegetables, legumes, and whole grains can help manage blood sugar levels. These foods can also keep you feeling full and satisfied.

4. **Opt for Lean Proteins**
- Choosing lean protein sources such as turkey, chicken, fish, and legumes can help balance your meals and manage your blood sugar levels.

5. **Stay Hydrated**
- Be sure to drink plenty of water throughout the day, especially if you are consuming foods with higher sodium content.

6. **Be Mindful of Alcohol Intake**
- If you choose to consume alcohol, do so in moderation and consider the impact on your blood sugar levels. Always drink responsibly and consider lower-sugar drink options.

7. **Engage in Physical Activity**
- Incorporating physical activity into your day, whether it's going for a walk or enjoying some active games with friends and family, can help

manage blood sugar and contribute to your overall well-being.

8. Choose Healthier Cooking Methods
- When preparing meals, opt for healthier cooking methods such as grilling, baking, or steaming instead of frying.

9. Enjoy Mindfully
- Be present and mindful while enjoying your meals. Take your time to savor each bite, and listen to your body's cues for hunger and fullness.

10. Seek Support
- Don't be afraid to seek support from friends and family. You can also consider sharing your dietary preferences or needs with the host to ensure that healthier options are available.

11. Pack Healthy Snacks
- If you're attending an event, consider bringing a few healthy snacks with you. This can help you manage your hunger and blood sugar levels throughout the day.

12. **Prioritize Rest**
- Getting adequate rest and managing stress is also important for overall health and well-being, which can also have an impact on blood sugar levels.

By being mindful of your choices and staying aware of your body's needs, you can fully enjoy festive occasions while managing diabetes and prioritizing your health and well-being. These tips can help you maintain balance, control your blood sugar levels, and fully enjoy the celebrations!

CHAPTER 7; KITCHEN TIPS AND SUBSTITUTIONS FOR DIABETES-FRIENDLY COOKING

7.1 Diabetes friendly substitutions for common ingredients

Making diabetes-friendly substitutions in your cooking and baking can help manage blood sugar levels and promote overall well-being. Here are some common ingredient substitutions for individuals managing diabetes:

1. **Sweeteners**
- Instead of sugar, consider using sugar substitutes such as stevia, monk fruit sweetener, erythritol, or xylitol. These sweeteners can provide sweetness without the significant impact on blood sugar levels.

2. **Flour**
- Instead of refined white flour, consider using almond flour, coconut flour, or flaxseed meal. These alternative flours offer more fiber and fewer carbohydrates than traditional refined flour.

3. **Cooking Oils**
- Instead of vegetable oil or shortening, opt for healthier oils such as olive oil, avocado oil, or coconut oil. These oils offer heart-healthy fats and can help manage cholesterol levels.

4. **Whole Grains**
- Instead of white rice or refined pasta, choose whole grains such as quinoa, brown rice, whole grain pasta, or bulgur. These whole grains offer more fiber and nutrients, which can have a more gradual impact on blood sugar levels.

5. **Dairy Products**
- Instead of full-fat dairy, opt for low-fat or non-fat dairy products to reduce saturated fat content. Alternatively, consider using plant-

based milk alternatives like almond milk, soy milk, or oat milk.

6. **Sweets and Desserts**
- Instead of traditional desserts, consider making fruit-based desserts or using sugar-free sweeteners in your baked goods. Using fresh fruits, sugar substitutes, and whole grains can help create delicious, diabetes-friendly desserts.

7. **Salty Snacks**
- Instead of high-sodium snacks, opt for unsalted nuts, seeds, or homemade popcorn with herbs and spices for flavor. Choosing snacks with less added salt can help manage blood pressure and overall cardiovascular health.

8. **Condiments**
- Instead of high-sugar sauces or dressings, consider making your own with fresh ingredients. You can use herbs, spices, and vinegar to create flavorful dressings and seasonings without excessive added sugars.

9. **Beverages**
- Instead of sugary drinks, choose water, sparkling water, or unsweetened tea. If you enjoy fruit juice, consider diluting it with water or choosing 100% fruit juice with no added sugars.

10. **Fruits and Vegetables**
- Instead of starchy vegetables, prioritize non-starchy vegetables such as leafy greens, broccoli, asparagus, and peppers. Also, balance fruit intake with portion control, and consider choosing whole fruits over fruit juices.

Making these diabetes-friendly ingredient substitutions can help support better blood sugar management, promote cardiovascular health, and contribute to overall well-being. It's important to consult with a healthcare professional or a registered dietitian before making significant changes to your diet, especially if you have specific dietary restrictions or health concerns.

7.2 : Cooking techniques for healthier meals

Using healthier cooking techniques can help retain nutrients and reduce the need for added fats and sugars, creating delicious and nutritious meals. Here are some cooking techniques to consider for healthier meal preparation:

1. Grilling

Grilling is a fantastic method for cooking lean proteins such as chicken, fish, and vegetables. It requires little to no added fats, as the high heat caramelizes food, producing a wonderful depth of flavor without excess oil.

2. Steaming

Steaming is a gentle cooking method that helps retain the natural flavors and nutrients in vegetables, fish, and grains. It's an especially good choice for preserving water-soluble vitamins that can be lost through boiling.

3. **Stir-Frying**

Stir-frying uses small amounts of heart-healthy oils and high heat, making it a quick and efficient way to cook vegetables and lean proteins. The fast-cooking time helps to maintain the texture and nutrients in the food.

4. **Roasting**

Roasting vegetables, lean cuts of meat, and fish is a wonderful way to intensify flavors while requiring minimal fat. It's a dry-heat cooking method that can bring out the natural sweetness and complexity of various ingredients.

5. **Baking**

Baking can be a healthier alternative to frying for preparing chicken, fish, and vegetables. It requires minimal oil and allows for a variety of seasoning options, helping to create flavorful dishes without the need for excessive fats.

6. **Poaching**

Poaching involves cooking delicate foods such as fish, chicken, or fruits in gently simmering liquid. It's a low-fat cooking technique that helps retain moisture and tenderness while infusing subtle flavors into the food.

7. **Sautéing**

Sautéing uses a small amount of heart-healthy oils over moderately high heat, making it a great technique for quickly cooking vegetables while preserving their texture and color.

8. **Broiling**

Broiling is a method that exposes food to direct radiant heat, resulting in a slightly crispy exterior while retaining moisture inside. It's a great option for lean cuts of meat and fish, as well as for quickly cooking vegetables.

9. **Sous Vide**

Sous vide involves vacuum-sealing food and cooking it in a precisely controlled water bath. This method helps retain nutrients and flavors while ensuring consistent, even cooking without requiring added fats.

10. **Raw Foods**

Incorporating raw foods, such as fresh salads and vegetable crudités, into your meal plans can offer nutrient-dense, low-calorie options that provide important enzymes and vitamins.

These cooking techniques not only help reduce the need for excessive fats and sugars, but they also allow you to retain the natural flavors and nutrients in your ingredients. By prioritizing these healthier cooking methods, you can transform your meals into delicious and nutritious culinary creations.

CHAPTER 8: RESOURCES AND FURTHER READING

8.1 Useful Websites and books for diabetes management

There are several reputable websites and books that offer valuable insights, guidance, and resources for diabetes management. Here are some helpful resources for diabetes management:

For Websites:

1. American Diabetes Association (ADA) - The ADA website provides a wealth of information on diabetes management, including tips for nutrition, physical activity, and a variety of helpful resources. (Website: [diabetes.org](https://www.diabetes.org/))

2. Centers for Disease Control and Prevention (CDC) - The CDC offers extensive information and resources on diabetes prevention, management, and healthy lifestyle habits.

(Website:
[cdc.gov/diabetes](https://www.cdc.gov/diabet
es/index.html))

3. Mayo Clinic - The Mayo Clinic website
features comprehensive information on
diabetes, including symptoms, causes,
treatments, and lifestyle strategies for
managing the condition. (Website:
[mayoclinic.org/diseases-
conditions/diabetes](https://www.mayoclinic.or
g/diseases-conditions/diabetes/symptoms-
causes/syc-20371444))

4. National Institute of Diabetes and Digestive
and Kidney Diseases (NIDDK) - NIDDK provides
valuable resources, research updates, and
information about diabetes and related
conditions. (Website: [niddk.nih.gov/health-
information/diabetes](https://www.niddk.nih.go
v/health-information/diabetes))

5. Diabetes UK - Diabetes UK offers a wide
range of resources, including guides on
diabetes management, lifestyle tips, and

personal stories from individuals living with diabetes. (Website: [diabetes.org.uk](https://www.diabetes.org.uk/))

For Books:

1. "**The End of Diabetes**: The Eat to Live Plan to Prevent and Reverse Diabetes" by Dr. Joel Fuhrman - This book provides a comprehensive guide to understanding and managing diabetes through nutritional strategies, lifestyle recommendations, and meal plans.

2. "**Think Like a Pancreas**: A Practical Guide to Managing Diabetes with Insulin" by Gary Scheiner - This book offers practical advice and strategies for insulin management, blood sugar control, and day-to-day management of diabetes.

3. "Diabetes Meal Planning and Nutrition for Dummies" by Toby Smithson, Alan L Rubin, and Consumer Dummies - This resource provides practical guidance on diabetes meal planning,

nutrition, and making healthier food choices for better blood sugar management.

4. **"Bright Spots & Landmines:** The Diabetes Guide I Wish Someone Had Handed Me" by Adam Brown - This insightful book offers practical tips, personal insights, and actionable strategies for living well with diabetes.

5. "**Dr. Neal Barnard's Program for Reversing Diabetes**: The Scientifically Proven System for Reversing Diabetes without Drugs" by Neal D. Barnard - Written by a renowned physician, this book offers science-based insights and practical guidance for managing and potentially reversing diabetes through lifestyle changes. These resources offer a wealth of information, guidance, and practical advice for individuals seeking to better understand and manage diabetes. From meal planning to lifestyle adjustments, these resources can offer valuable support and insights. Always consult with a healthcare professional for personalized advice and guidance tailored to your specific health needs.

8.2 Kitchen tools for diabetes friendly cooking

When it comes to diabetes-friendly cooking, having the right kitchen tools can make meal preparation easier, from portion control to healthier cooking methods. Here are several kitchen tools that can be particularly useful for diabetes-friendly cooking:

1. **Food Scale:**
Accurately measuring portion sizes and ingredient quantities is essential for diabetes management. A digital food scale can help ensure precise measurements and better control over carbohydrate intake.

2. **Measuring Cups and Spoons:**
Measuring cups and spoons are essential for portion control and accurate measurement of ingredients when preparing meals, especially for baked goods and cooking from recipes.

3. **Steamer Basket:**

A steamer basket enables the gentle cooking of vegetables, fish, and other foods, helping to retain moisture, nutrients, and natural flavors without the need for added fats.

4. **Non-Stick Cookware:**

Non-stick cookware requires less oil for cooking, making it ideal for preparing healthier meals with minimized added fats.

5. **Grilling Pan or Grill:**

Grilling pans and outdoor grills are great for cooking lean proteins and vegetables, allowing for delicious, low-fat meals without the need for excessive oil.

6. **Vegetable Spiralizer:**

A vegetable spiralizer can be used to turn vegetables such as zucchini, carrots, or sweet potatoes into low-carb alternatives to pasta, providing more options for diabetes-friendly meal choices.

7. **Blender or Food Processor:**
Blenders and food processors are useful for making nutritious smoothies, homemade sauces, soups, and dips using whole, fresh ingredients.

8. **Air Fryer:**
An air fryer can create crispy and flavorful foods using a minimal amount of oil, offering a healthier cooking alternative to traditional deep frying.

9. **Instant Pot or Electric Pressure Cooker:**
These versatile appliances can speed up cooking times while preserving the natural flavors and nutrients of ingredients, making meal preparation more efficient.

10. **Salad Spinner:**
A salad spinner makes it easy to wash and dry leafy greens and vegetables, ensuring that you have fresh and clean produce for salads and other dishes.

11. **Herb Mill or Herb Scissors:**

Fresh herbs can add flavor to dishes without the need for added sugars or excess fats. Herb mills or scissors make it easier to finely chop or shred herbs for seasoning.

12. **Citrus Juicer:**

Freshly squeezed citrus juice can provide a burst of flavor to dishes, marinades, and dressings without added sugars or processed ingredients.

Having these kitchen tools on hand can make diabetes-friendly meal preparation more convenient and enjoyable, offering the opportunity to create delicious and nutritious dishes while supporting blood sugar management and overall health.

www.ingramcontent.com/pod-product-compliance
Lightning Source LLC
Chambersburg PA
CBHW060945260726
48661CB00005B/1761